BEING WELL

~ deciding on your health and healing ~

ISBN 978-1-8383550-8-1

© Cover Design Lisa Gentle

Keekoo Publications

www.richardgentle.co.uk

First Edition 2015

Revised Edition 2024

Foreword

Why are so many people ill? Science, doctors, nutritionists, clinicians, the pharmaceutical industry, and other 'experts' would like us to believe that illness is going to affect all of us and at least half of us can pretty much expect to get cancer of one form or another in our lifetime!

But what if illness is only the physical manifestation of our beliefs, psychology, feelings, and expectations? What if all the marketing and advertising of illness is the very thing that is increasing it?

Although much has been said about physical symptoms only being the outward manifestation of inner difficulties, this booklet attempts to go deeper. If you have a persistent or terminal illness, it may be challenging for you to read this booklet at first – but be assured that the truth it contains could change your life... or even cure you.

Contents

Our relationship with health and illness

This book may be controversial in places and possibly disquieting for some. However, just because it puts forward views that contradict society's strongly held cultural and personal beliefs about health and illness this shouldn't be a reason to condemn alternative truth that must be expressed.

Cancer is going to be mentioned in this book, but not in the usual way. No one is denying that it can be awful or debilitating, but I will be straight-talking about some of its origins; it's 'oh dear, ain't it awful' public sycophantic sentimentality; and applause for pundits who raise money for band-wagon research by shaming the fit and well into parting with their cash out of fear, embarrassment, coercion, and emotional blackmail, at every opportunity. You want a cure? I will offer you a cure for free – but it's up to you whether you can accept it or not.

1. A natural state of good health

Philosophical and 'spiritual teachers' (Gurus) have said for centuries that our natural state of being is one of health. I have to admit, I really didn't understand the sentiment when I first came across it, since around me were people with all manner of ailments and health-related incapacities. If we should all be healthy – why aren't we?

If this does not make sense – that our natural state is one of good health – then obviously we are missing something. We must look deeper and probably from a different perspective.

2. Science acknowledges only a physical universe

Western society has decided that only science can save its world from impending doom. Put on a white coat and some glasses and everyone will take your words seriously. Stick letters before or after your name and you become a knowledgeable authority and trustworthy advocate of how things really are. After all, you have 'tested' things and reached strong conclusions based on those resultant 'facts'.

But, why do we so readily believe what we are told? Is it that we are not interested in questioning? Do other people know more about us than we do? Is it that we assume someone of seemingly more importance than our self must know the answers? Does wearing a uniform and having a university education equate to an unquestionable knowledge beyond our own possibility for individual comprehension? Or do we accept narrow formal qualifications, peer-review status, and public celebrity, as the only marks of true validity?

We have to appreciate that we are experiencing a physical realm – one of many realms available to us as energetic [soul] entities – and as such, we are here to develop our skills and understanding of this realm and how we contribute to its form and identity through our conscious beliefs, thoughts and actions.

Science likes to prove through observation and repeatable experiments. However, even scientists are now coming to accept that the quantum universe is more about probable outcomes than neatly packaged, predictable, or isolated events of chance. Despite this, there is still a refusal to step away from mainstream methodologies and accept that some things appear that cannot be tested or repeated under lab conditions. We can only go so far with treating, or finding solutions for, physical symptoms, when we only look for their physical causes and not their psycho-emotional and vibrational connections.

Furthermore, funding for research is naturally aimed at the most popular and pressing causes and because of this, many researchers will apply for grants in relation to where the highest funding is likely to be forthcoming, rather than where it is not. In the case of Cancer Research, everyone involved in raising money for finding cures is onto a winner, because there are as many variants as there are common colds – and who has yet found a cure-all for those?

3. Sex and a lemon

In some of my previous books, I give a couple of examples of how our thoughts can affect our physical body chemistry. The first example is to imagine cutting the top off a fresh lemon and then sinking your teeth into the sour flesh inside. The second example is to think of something sexual that 'turns you on' and notice the responses this has in your body.

So, what's the point of that? Well, if two simple thoughts can create such an effect on your body, why would you suppose that other thoughts don't also affect your body chemistry? And if you change your body chemistry, and it creates imbalances, you are very likely going to see and experience physical results. Furthermore, as you will come to appreciate later, the beliefs that you hold about your life and the world you experience will determine the very nature and experience of any dis-ease that you encounter. This is one reason why two people could have the same diagnosis of physical symptoms, yet respond quite differently in their ability to heal – or not.

4. Water

Japanese researcher, Masaru Emoto[1] (1943-2014) became internationally famous after publishing his observations on frozen water crystals. He wrote a number of books containing the title of 'Messages from Water' where he demonstrated how projected emotion through words and music directly affected the crystalline structures in positive or negative ways. If you extrapolate these findings, it doesn't take a big leap of the imagination to realise, given that our bodies are over 50% water, our thoughts and what we absorb from the 'noise' around us, together with our internal chatter or 'self-talk'[2], can very likely affect our physical body chemistry.

5. Food and drink

There used to be a saying: 'You are what you eat.' Many people do indeed believe this – particularly those who have adopted sensitivity or experience allergic reactions to certain foods and drinks, or their ingredients – but its wider implication is that the quality of our food has a positive or negative effect on our physical and mental well-being. Consider for example, the Gerson Therapy[3], where organic juicing of fruit and vegetables has been shown to work healing wonders for many, once terminally ill, people.

Of course, like everything else about our experience of reality, what we believe about our food becomes true to us individually. Contrary to the beliefs of many, you can pretty much eat whatever you want to eat. However, there is a caveat to this statement. If at some level you believe that something is of detriment to you, then regardless of its perceived value, it is going to affect you in negative ways. Likewise, if 'good food' is not palatable to you, and you really don't enjoy eating it, then that can't be doing you much good either. I'm sorry, but the old adage of 'if it [the medicine or suggested help] hurts or tastes bad – it must be good for you!' doesn't wash with me. Moderation in all things, is better.

6. Medication

In addition to our thoughts, feelings, and consumption of food and drink, one of the biggest effects on our bodies is commercial medication. It's almost a standing joke, that when we take a pill for one thing, very often we have to take another pill to counter some side-effects of the first pill – until eventually, and particularly as we get older, we are reliant on a balancing act between 24 or more pills a day to maintain our ability to function.

Also, reaching for the medicine cabinet as our first choice of health correction is not giving the body an opportunity to make many of the corrections that it is naturally able to perform. One reason for our action is our need to resolve things fast – the quick fix in a work-time-focused world.

If the ailment is more than a headache, we will often visit our local GP[4] (Doctor) – although, in the UK, it is usually women more than men who take up this option.[5] But, whichever way you look at it, there is a sense of devolved responsibility for one's own wellbeing, or a perceived inability to manage our own health with any confidence. Although, it has to be acknowledged, that more of us check the Internet for possible solutions to our symptoms, these days.

Treatments then received, by way of formalised medication, often deal with one specific symptom, and little questioning is done into the possible root causes and even less when it comes to suggesting non-medical remedies. Because our bodies are holistic and not compartmentalised, medication aimed at one thing could throw another part of us into some imbalance requiring additional compensation from our body organism.

7. The law of attraction

At its simplest, the Law of Attraction states that what you regularly focus your attention on is drawn towards you like a magnet. In other words, what you focus on you create more of. Because the universe does not differentiate between something being 'good' or 'bad', the focus on anything deemed 'good' or 'bad' by an individual, group, or culture, will be interpreted through Law of Attraction as something desired. So focusing on something unwanted has similar pulling power to focusing on something desired. However, because [for many] feelings of discomfort often trigger thoughts that seem to carry greater emotional strength, the power to attract our 'negative' experiences seems more prevalent.

You experience the reality that you create and as Seth, (a non-physical energy personality)[6] says: we all create our own experiences from the beliefs we hold about reality. Notice here that we talk about 'beliefs we hold about reality' and not that our beliefs are reality. Sure, the feedback we appear to receive through living in reality could be deemed as evidence for our beliefs being correct. However, it doesn't really work this way... and like many things in life, the opposite of what we appear to notice is often closer to a truth of what is really occurring.

8. Fear-based health marketing

It is a sad fact, for many living in consumer-driven societies around the world, that fear is a great motivator to taking 'preventative action' – often for no actually present reason. Everything from: securing our homes, to insuring ourselves against all manner of potential calamities. Top of the bill at present, are a plethora of health-related things we must worry about and keep checking for evidence of – until we can actually find we have them. The two worst [UK] culprits are cancer and dental care. If you take television marketing alone, there must be hundreds of commercials shown every day that mention various forms of cancer, tooth decay, or gum disease. This constant bombardment against the human psyche is not one of care – it is one of recruitment. Not to mention the cost of this marketing, which some might think could be better spent in helpful research.

If you constantly send out negative and worrying messages to people, they start to be concerned that they are likely to witness mirrored circumstances in their own lives. By 'Law of Attraction'[7] alone, we attract more of what we focus our attention on. We see this, not only in areas of health but, also in areas of violence and sexual deviancy or abuse (the preferred descriptors of society's media protagonists).

Because of the way our wellbeing is marketed, it's easy to take the cynical view that this approach is more about raising money to keep people and industries in employment and profit, than it is to promote a well-balanced and healthy population.

The focus on negative messages

'Smoking Kills' is a message we are all familiar with. Unfortunately, society's predilection for 'shock and awe' over positive reinforcement really is not helpful. We think that by shouting against, or fighting everything, we can stir people to action. Sadly, the originators of these negative campaigns base them on fear and ignorance, rather than hope. Every time a smoker sees a packet with 'smoking kills', it simply says 'tough shit mate – you're going to die!' The individual may wish they did not smoke, but the habit is powerful – or even, dare I say it, enjoyed. A more helpful message might be: 'Healthier not to smoke' or something similar. Surely this is a message of positive suggestion and much more in line with the desired outcome of all concerned – with the exception of the tobacco manufacturers, of course.

I have quoted Mother Teresa many times in my books as saying: *"I will never attend an anti-war rally; if you have a peace rally, invite me."* She knew that so long as the word 'war' was used, the focus would still include the vibration of war and through the Law of Attraction, and the concern and fear of war, the very thing we did not want, would be perpetuated. A focus on peace and love can only produce a peace and love vibration and therefore attract more of the same.

It is similar when voting for Political leadership – Governments. The more that people do not want a particular party or leader to gain office, the more likely it is that those people you do not want will win their election. All of your anxiety and focus is on those people. In a Law of Attraction universe, your message is not, 'keep them out!' it is, 'let them in!'

What we must do therefore, is focus more of our attention on the outcomes we would like to experience and less on the outcomes that we fear will happen. Of course, for most of us, seeing something different to what appears to be evidently in front of us is not something that comes naturally or easily.

9. The direction of focus

It has always amazed me that almost all of the money collected for Cancer Research is officially designated to 'finding cures'. You may not realise it, but quite a number of people get remission from cancer[8] and go on to lead normal healthy lives – without the use of chemotherapy or other medical interventions. How about channelling some funding to research the causes behind these remissions?

There have been a number of television programmes devoted to alternative cancer treatments and cures over the years and most of those have been quickly pilloried by the establishment. Documentaries that proclaim to be impartial have used filming techniques with subtle lighting effects and sound tracks to belittle views that might draw criticism of the programme makers. Disparaging comments have been wrapped in snide humour and those advocating any form of easily available natural cure have been labelled as selling 'snake oil'[9].

Furthermore, there is a corporate interest in not finding natural or free cures to major diseases. There is a vested interest by all those who can gain financially, create job opportunities and expand businesses – particularly those in the drug, pharmaceutical or medical devices industries. Free cures from some plant or other, at the bottom of someone's garden, is not on the agenda for consideration.

10. Opposites

As touched on earlier, many things in our physical experience are quite opposite to what we believe them to be. Most people experience a world that is outside of them, seemingly affecting how they feel moment to moment. However, the world you experience 'out there' is only feedback for the 'inner world' you create with your emotional thoughts and feelings – and any thought or feeling you have is based solely upon a belief that you hold as true in your experience. External experience reflected back, reinforces inner beliefs of being right. This is cumulative reinforcement – sometimes referred to as 'confirmation bias.'

As you focus your thoughts with emotion, you gradually affect the way you respond to those thoughts, ideas, and developing beliefs. This forms a vibrational frequency signature that emanates from you electromagnetically[10] to interface with universal consciousness, or as Seth[11] calls it, 'All That Is'. This emanation becomes your principal attractor for all things and events that occur in your life and enables you to objectify apparently exterior things as having physical substance. As you begin to focus your thoughts and feelings differently and with consistency, you can alter this emanation – either for personal benefit, or detriment, to your wellbeing. Ideally, your progressive understanding of the universal principles will help you to attract more beneficial outcomes – challenging at first, but not impossible. As an extra observation, I'd suggest that those people who do not 'over think' things too much, will have more success than those who do.

11. Pressure on societies

Large numbers of people experience an ever-complex and fast-paced world, where fitting in, working in pressurised environments, or simply feeling they are 'fighting for survival', becomes paramount to their individual and collective focus. This type of stress causes quite a lot of inner upset and perhaps it is not realised how this can affect the types of increasingly new and complex diseases and ailments now experienced. We cannot easily foretell how some emotional upsets are going to manifest in our physical experiences.

12. Beliefs about reality

The statement that our individual beliefs colour our experience is fundamental to the life we lead. To keep things simple, let me focus on the life we lead in the physical reality of our world as we perceive it and en masse, understand it. We all experience a physical life and we all experience an emotional life. What few of us will accept is a deeper connection between the two – in an opposite way around way to what we are used to accepting.

As stated earlier, it is all about our beliefs. Take any emotion that you are experiencing right now and ask yourself: 'Why do I feel this way?' You can be sure that it is connected to a belief you hold about something. Then ask yourself: Is this belief I hold, true? Really take some time to consider your responses. It is most likely too, that many of the beliefs you hold come from the misunderstanding, or the fear, of something. But consider Mark Twain's[12] famous quote: *"I've had a lot of worries in my life, most of which never happened."*

13. The emotional connection

Having now read through some of the previous sections, we can begin to link things together to discover more about the nature of our health, both as individuals, groups, societies, and cultures. Perhaps the easiest one to start with is the last – cultural beliefs.

We all grow up in an atmosphere of beliefs from those around us. As an individual, one naturally accepts varying levels of those beliefs, mostly without question and often in subliminal ways. For example, children absorb much more information than we give them credit for, when learning about their environments and the objectified things and people that come into their sphere of notice, or affect their sense of wellbeing. As we gain in experience and age, some of our beliefs are clearly accepted as fact while others may raise questions that we either explore further, or dismiss as anomalies we don't have time for, or resonate with.

We develop our own filing boxes for 'true', 'false', 'don't know', and 'don't care'. The trouble is the 'don't know' box is, more often than not, kicked under the bed to be conveniently ignored, where it simply gathers dust.

Because those before our arrival have already made decisions about some of their beliefs collectively, their culture broadly accepts a core of understanding to be a truth about the reality they experience together. A sub-set of these beliefs is held by families and individuals, who both 'accept' and live by 'the rules' associated with those beliefs. However, many of those beliefs are no longer consciously held in the active mind – that is to say, the individual is not thinking about beliefs as a number one priority for daily functioning.

By analogy, once you learn to drive a manual car, you do not consciously think about how to change gear, use the clutch or balance the accelerator, each time you go anywhere. The action is automatic and autonomic[13]. Holding the belief consciously, about how the gear-changing works, is no longer necessary – it goes without saying that the process of changing gear is a standard truth about that particular reality of driving a geared vehicle. The belief needs no questioning because it is a fact associated with a known and quantifiable activity and action – the same as moving a limb or walking about.

So how can this be applied to health? Well, if you live in a culture that believes that colds can be passed on from person to person via airborne sneezes containing 'viruses', then your expectation for 'catching' a cold in these circumstances is strong. It is a belief that does not require examination or questioning. Everyone [now] knows that colds can be passed on to others in this way. But is it actually true for everyone? There are many people who never catch colds in this way. They are simply unconcerned when someone sneezes in their presence. Perhaps it is not something that has been mentioned by others, or even concerns someone. Perhaps the person sneezing actually does not have any cold or ailments that could be spread – maybe it was just dust or a change in the lighting conditions that triggered the sneezing response. The point here is that a concern for something derives from a [fear] belief held about it. This stimulates an emotional response that focuses the mind's thoughts in one direction – that of concern for personal wellbeing. Consider some of these:

Don't pick food up that you've just dropped on the floor. Why not? Because the floor is dirty and germs may get on the food and then you will be ill.

Don't get cold or wet in the rain and don't get cold after washing your hair, because you might catch a cold. Why? Doctor Joshi[14] says: *"Getting a cold from going out in the cold or after washing your hair is a myth. Colds are common. If the virus[15] is already there and then you go out with wet hair and develop symptoms, it's common to think that is what caused it."*

Take Vitamin C to stop or cure a cold. Why? Dr Joshi says, *"Research has found no evidence that vitamin C prevents colds."* (But I bet that won't stop people taking Vitamin C to try and alleviate colds).[16]

Fluoride is good for teeth. Is it? And it prevents decay. Does it? And it should be put in drinking water to stem tooth decay in children. Really? I do not intend to go into this too much, but there is plenty of information on the Internet and a campaign for preventing the use of Fluoride in water has been running since 1947[17]. Suffice to say, Fluoride for 'fighting tooth decay' is another popular (but false) myth firmly entrenched in many of our belief systems.[18]

The Titanic[19] hit an iceberg and sank. Did it? Some research has suggested that it was very likely that coal caught fire in the bunkers close to the massive boilers used to generate power through steam. An explosion from coal gas could have ripped a hole in the ship, or the heat from bunker coal fires could have damaged and warped important bulkheads. Evidence of this may have been later hull reinforcement – suggesting a problem of structural integrity covered up. Perhaps hitting an iceberg was the final straw, so-to-speak. However, popular myth will always tend to endure as truth.

Hopefully, you can begin to see how accepted beliefs create thoughts in your mind, which in turn stimulate an emotional response, which then has a physical effect on the way your body starts to feel.

14. Background, history and blame

One thing many people refuse to do is take any responsibility for the predicaments they find themselves in when it comes to health. Seth[20] offers many valuable insights into our wellbeing regarding personal health and here is a great one:

"Each thought has a result, in your terms. The same kind of thought, habitually repeated, will seem to have a more or less permanent effect. If you like the effect then you seldom examine the thought. If you find yourself assailed by physical difficulties, however, you begin to wonder what is wrong.

"Sometimes you blame others, your own background, or a previous life – if you accept reincarnation. You may hold God or the Devil responsible, or you may simply say, 'That is life' and accept the negative experience as a necessary portion of your lot.

"You may finally come to a half-understanding of the nature of reality and wail, 'I believe that I have caused these ill effects, but I find myself unable to reverse them.'

"If this is the case, then regardless of what you have told yourself thus far, you still do not believe that you are the creator of your own experience. As soon as you recognize this fact you can begin at once to alter those conditions that cause you dismay or dissatisfaction.

"No one forces you to think in any particular manner. In the past you may have learned to consider things pessimistically. You may believe that pessimism is more realistic than optimism. You may even suppose, and many do, that sorrow is ennobling, a sign of deep spiritualism, a mark of apartness, a necessary mental garb of saints and poets. Nothing could be further from the truth."[21]

So keep reaching for a better thought. Know that it is possible to use your thoughts to change any belief that causes a negative emotional response. However, this does take persistent and regular practice.

15. Changing beliefs

Some beliefs may seem easier to change than others, although one thing they all have in common is that they are based on personal experiences from the repetition of supporting evidence (or perceived continuing evidence) *in the personal reality of the individual.* That last part is very important to remember. The reality you experience is your own – no one else's. This is useful as your starting point because if your reality is personal to you, then you have power over its truth in your experience. No one can impose their version of reality on you, unless you have vibrational resonance[22] to that version of reality.

Abraham[23] (a channelled collective of teachers) says: *"You have power of influence, but you cannot create in the experience of another."*

Abraham also says of those who witness illness in others: *"When you believe in their wellness, even when they don't, your influence is stronger."*

And when a person asks from a place of focused determination, Abraham adds: *"Their asking is superseding any doubt or belief they've ever had, so, for a moment, they quantum leap."*

16. Vibrational matching

"You can't be something you don't have and be a vibrational match to it." – Abraham[24]

'Vibrational resonance' or 'matching' can be simply described in two analogous ways: A tuning fork and a radio.

Musicians may sometimes use a tuning fork[25] to gain a perfect pitch for their instrument or voice. Once there is no difference in tone between the noise from the fork and the voice, or a string on a guitar, then both are in tune with each other and only one harmonic sound pitch can be heard.

If you have a radio, you know that there are many stations to choose from, but you also know that you only hear one station at a time (when you tune the radio to a clear broadcast frequency). Although you may listen to only one channel, you are aware that there are other channels that exist simultaneously, but at different frequencies that you are not at present tuned to. In order to experience a different channel, you have to re-tune to that frequency.

In terms of your own personhood, re-focusing your thoughts has similarities to the radio analogy. You tend to follow emotionally, where your thoughts lead you. A thought that seems to carry more emotion – positive or negative – also seems to gain strength, momentum, and clarity. However, unlike a radio, where you can simply re-tune in an instant, our mental ability to re-tune can be obstinate – preferring to doggedly hold on to the station we are experiencing.

Feeling upset about something often causes our re-tuning wheel to stick solid. And if we do manage to momentarily tune into a different thought, very quickly it springs back to the focus that seems to have the greatest draw for us.

17. Why is it so hard to re-focus?

The difference between the radio and our mind is that the radio carries no emotional attachment to the station it is tuned to. We, on the other hand, seem to have vested interests in our thoughts – and a need to react to the emotions seemingly activated by them. Feelings of annoyance, anger, frustration, injustice, blame, etc., to mention only a few of the most common, are typically the things that hold our focus and stop us re-tuning. The last one, 'blame', is a particular favourite. Before we can 'let go' or re-focus, someone has to be accountable for what has happened; what I've lost; what I feel, etc. Finding something, or someone, to blame for our discomfort absolves us of any further responsibility. 'No need to feel involvement anymore – it was someone else's fault. It was nothing to do with me. I am vindicated.' A family example of this might be: Dad shouts at Mum; Mum shouts at their child; and the child kicks the cat. Each, in turn, passing on their frustration and not realising their part in the creation of their event, experience and emotion.

18. Beliefs about time

Something else that will benefit our health and healing recovery is a re-evaluation of the nature of time. Time, in our world, has become our main governor of activity, progression and expectation for due outcomes. We divide our lives by intervals and segments – daily activity to general life expectancy. We see progression as a series of linear events unfolding over a finite time period – one thing leading to another.

A sense of time allows us to consider our options and firm up our thoughts and ideas. A sense of a past gives us a feeling of evolution and reflection. A sense of our present enables us to live in the moment and make conscious changes for our future. And a sense of a future helps us to imagine something that we might like to experience (or fear) in our next moments of 'now'.

But the reality of our linear time is that it does not exist. What we have is what Seth[26] calls a 'spacious present'[27]. From this place, we are able to simultaneously draw on all 'past' and 'future' qualities of our 'multidimensional personality'[28] and bring them together in what he terms 'the moment point'[29] – that which we choose to experience in our 'now'.

If this is indeed the case, then spontaneous healing should be possible. Of course, it quickly becomes 'impossible' once we apply our current beliefs about our rational reality to the mix.

You might say, with incredulity: 'It took this amount of time to reach my state of ill-health, so how can it not take a reasonable period of time to recover?'

Here's something to think about. When you have a cold, with a running nose, how often do you have to reach for another tissue? Isn't it amazing how you can blow your nose dry and yet seconds later, it needs blowing again. How can the body produce that much activity so rapidly?

At first, you may see no relevance in that last observation to what is being discussed in relation to health and healing. However, if your body has the ability to produce something at that speed, then surely it could be equally capable of getting you better at similar speeds. All you have to do is find something that activates this process.

19. Memories and time

Believe it or not, we cannot rely on our memories – particularly those involving others. We can only form agreements with those whom we share relationships of our own making.

If you think about it, an individual's memories of events are very personal and coloured by the emotions felt at the time about the experiences, coupled with the beliefs held now. It is actually possible to change any aspect of your past from your present moment. Simply choose which bits of your past you want to focus on and see them without judgement or concern. If you remember something unhappy, start to search for the moments that were the opposite – happy… or at least lighter. With practice, you can bring the most positive feelings into your present – changing your feelings about certain past events to more positive and helpful vibrations. You can even converse with your younger self and offer reassurances.

If this isn't enough to convince you about memories, ask friends or family to recount past events that you all shared together and see how many variations arise from what was remembered and what was not.

So what of the future? Whatever you are thinking most strongly about now, is what you are projecting forward. The best way to see your future is to imagine living the experiences you want to be having in your 'now' moment. This takes practice because you have to ignore patterns of resistance and the 'already physically manifested' life you are witnessing around you.

20. Beliefs about health

It is important to trust your body in knowing that you will always be in good health, or at the very least, able to recover from any illness, ailment, or physical affliction that seems to befall you.

If you have always suffered from poor health, this may seem to be an unhelpful statement for me to launch in your direction. I might as well have said, 'Come on... stop moping around... pick yourself up and just get better.' It's easy for someone who can already do something with ease, to wonder why everyone else has so much difficulty doing the same. I could cite many instances in my own life where others who have mastered what, at times, I consider to be my failings or impossible impasses, have said similarly to me. It doesn't exactly endear you to someone, does it? However, we must continue to explore this sense of 'knowing you can be healthy' more fully.

Let us begin with personal honesty. Within the confined privacy of your own thoughts, can you answer the following questions?

- Does my illness serve me in any way?
- Is there something I do not want to do which illness excuses me from?

- Could any of the thoughts or beliefs I hold, manifest themselves into the physical symptoms I am experiencing?
- Do I have any conflicting feelings about anything?
- Do I feel guilty about something?
- Do I feel I deserve punishment?
- Am I upset about someone or something, but feel unable to say or do anything about him, her, or it?
- Do I regularly use expressions such as: 'I feel the weight of the world is on my shoulders'; or 'so and so is a pain in the butt'; or 'it gives me a headache just thinking about it.'?

The above are just a few things you might consider, but learn to look for others if none of these provide relevant answers. Look for any symbolism associated with your illness, such as the last examples noted in the list.

21. The advantages of being ill

I realised a long time ago, that illness or injury provides us with the only legitimate excuse not to do something. It can also provide a conduit for love and attention for both the young and the elderly and particularly those who live alone without regular personal interactions with people, by which I mean, actually having someone visit or spend time with them in the same locality – not just speaking over the phone or via a video app.

Consider an occasion when you don't feel like going to work. Generally speaking, you can't call in and say: 'You know what? I don't feel like doing anything today.' It's certainly a way to attract a reprimand. On the other hand, calling in with Flu or food poisoning, usually elicits a response of: 'Oh dear – poor you. I do hope you feel better soon. Just relax and come in as soon as you feel well enough.'

A child learns early on that crying gets fast attention more effectively than tugging at a parent's sleeve. A lonely person discovers that inability to function brings relatives to the door much faster than phoning to arrange a date in someone's busy diary.

When we discover that illness produces 'rewards', it's easy to continue using it. However, there often comes a time when feigning illness actually becomes real illness that is difficult to shift. When this happens, we can lose control of our crutch and it becomes our burden. As we see and feel the evidence of our condition, we only see and feel our condition more. It consumes our focus and affects every decision we make about our daily life. Although we then wish to feel better, we believe in the futility of getting well again for all sorts of new reasons – most based on cultural, medical expectations that take a rational approach in substantiating their proof of futility. We now become a self-proclaimed victim, refusing to take any self-responsibility that could improve our lot.

22. Healing without change

During my time working with people and their health, one thing became very apparent. Unless the patient changes his or her behaviour[30], that is to say, the circumstances that caused the problem in the first place, any healing received is going to be of limited value and may only result in a temporary or partial improvement in the reported condition. In many ways, one could say the same about taking medications – only the symptoms are often further deadened to hide, rather than cure, the causes. To put things another way, if you have arm ache and it came about through sitting awkwardly at the computer, and you then have some healing, which takes away the pain, it's not helpful to return to your computer and sit in the same position again. Although that seems to be a somewhat obvious example, the principle is the same when the condition is of emotional origin.[31] This is where things can become more complex, since locating the root cause may be different to what you think it could be. You may literally have to do some soul-searching. For example, a feeling of lack may at first seem connected to financial circumstances, but on further investigation may come from being refused something as a child which you interpreted as being unworthy or un-loveable – that you cannot receive what you feel you need.

If you do request help from a healer, bear in mind that healing with the help of another is a collaborative process where both parties need to be on the same side. For fastest results, you and the healer have to see you as well, no matter what appears to be information to the contrary. A good healer will give you positive encouragement and when he or she is away from you, will continue to imagine your improvement. A good patient will believe in the possibility of improvement and start to look for signs of positive change. He, she, they, will expect to get better and this act alone will activate powerful resources in the mind and body to promote wellness.

23. The problem with cause and effect, karma, and beliefs about linear time

We are generally brought up to accept the Newtonian[32] discovery that for every action there is an equal and opposite reaction. Whilst this was Newton's Third Law of Motion[33] in a physical universe, it was not intended to be a reflection of general 'cause and effect', as in, 'what goes around comes around', used in a human and cultural context. Indeed, most westerners gained their understanding of such an idea from what eastern cultures refer to as karma – suggesting that not only do people gain 'good' or 'bad' karma, but that this can extend across [reincarnational[34]] lifetimes – requiring atonement when the balance is deemed to be weighted negatively. Unfortunately, it has also been used to justify all manner of human situations and conditions from extreme wealth and good fortune to abject poverty and lowly victimhood.

If time is not what we perceive it to be – a series of linear events of past, present and future – then Seth's description of a 'spacious present' leaves us in something of a quandary, since karma and the so-called law of cause and effect, cannot exist.

Seth says:

"The cause and effect theory being the result of continuity holds no water. When the spacious present is understood, with its attributes of spontaneity, then the cause and effect theory will fall."

Interestingly, like many things we experience, the absence of our acknowledgement or understanding of a 'spacious present' does not prevent us from having a life experience – in the same way that moving from a Newtonian universe to a Quantum universe[35] didn't prevent us from having a life experience either. We can still function, despite not knowing or understanding the bigger picture.

However, it seems that we are really missing out if we do not begin to consider that we have something more available to us, to enhance our life experience.

Seth goes on to say:

"You are in the spacious present now. You were in the spacious present in your yesterday and you will not have travelled through it in your tomorrow, or eons of tomorrows."

Lynda madden Dahl[36] offers her own commentary on this:

"Any other time scheme used by consciousness is camouflage constructed within the spacious present. And that's because, as Seth reminds us, in actuality there is only a spacious present.

"In fact, Seth says, 'there is no place to go. It is also true to say there are as many places to go as you wish to find.'

"Seth continues that, 'Identity, like action, is a dimension of existence.' And 'The reality of an identity exists within the action.'

"Realities are a part of identity/action. Which, when dropped to the bottom line, says I have my reality and you have yours, but we do not share realities per

se, because I'm within my identity (as we learned in the three dilemmas)[37] and you are within yours."

In some ways, this is probably the most difficult section of this booklet to get one's head around. Going off at a slight tangent to perhaps help the explanations thus far, think of the times you dream in your sleep. You can play out a whole time period, travelling all over the place and meeting others – all without moving from your bed. If you do not believe that you experience dreaming, another example might be immersive gaming.[38] You can travel all over the place and reach new levels of experience – all from the chair in your room.

So, returning to our previous discourse, if you extrapolate this view further, how can you become ill from an external source if no one, other than you, has direct access to your identity and, because linear time is illusory, how can an illness evolve over time?

In the spacious present, we can bring into being anything we select from our focus, whether it is past, present, or future. We can live in the 'moment point' of 'now' and by holding onto any aspect of our manifesting, appear to take it with us through a sense of linear time. If on the other hand, we had the mental discipline to completely let go of one thing and focus on another, we might start to spontaneously change in our 'moment point'.

24. Changing beliefs about illness

Changing our belief about something isn't simply a new state of denial. However, it is a new way of considering our situation. Many times, we feel powerless – particularly when we don't understand, or feel we do not have access to, the right knowledge. This is why we so often abdicate personal responsibility to other people 'more expert' than we are. However, just because we do not understand Latin, does not mean we cannot communicate. In the same way, just because we are not doctors, does not mean we cannot imagine what it would feel like if we were healthy again. If you need another example, you do not need to know every functional detail of how the engine works to drive a car – although it obviously helps to have some practice driving.

The important thing to consider here is you do not need to understand all of the intricate workings of your body to effect an improvement. All you have to do is focus your thoughts and attention on gaining an improvement. I would personally go one stage further than this and 'decide to be well'. Okay, at first this might seem ridiculous, but please give it a go – at least once or twice each day – regardless of what may seem to be apparent in any observation to the contrary. (Later in this book, I will give you a few simple self-healing exercises that you can try).

If it helps you to imagine or focus on something positive, create your own ritual. Play at it like a child – believe in magic and miracles. Make, buy, or find, a special object that you can imbue with 'special powers'. Do anything that changes your low feeling to something more hopeful.

Make some new decisions. Decide that you are going to recover – regardless of what anyone else has told you. Doctors seem to pride themselves in dishing out finite or worst-case scenarios. As someone [not sure who] once commented: 'If you're told that something is 'incurable', think of it instead as 'curable from within'.' The truth is medical research does not have all the answers. Doctors are people too – doing the best they can with what they know, understand, and have come to believe in their own experience. However, they often underestimate their power to counter healing through careless or, quite frankly, ill-considered remarks (pun accepted). There is a well-known situation called 'the placebo effect', where a confident suggestion by an authoritative person can trigger a positive belief. Usually, this is achieved in trials of pills, where none of the patients are told which of them are being prescribed actual medication. Of course, this can work in the opposite way if you tell the patients that some of them are going to be given poison.

25. A few health-related quotes from Seth

"Any physical ailment is symbolic of an inner reality or statement. Your entire life is a statement in physical terms, written upon time as you understand it."

~

"You must learn, of course, what the various symbols mean in your own life, and how to translate their meaning.[39]

"To do so, you must first of all remind yourself frequently that the physical condition IS symbolic − not a permanent condition. Then you must look within yourself for the inner actuality represented by the symbol.

"This same process can be followed regardless of the nature of the problem, or of your challenge."

~

"Quite literally, the 'inner self' forms the body by magically transforming thoughts and emotions into physical counterparts. You grow the body. Its condition perfectly mirrors your subjective state at any given time. Using atoms and molecules, you build your body, forming basic elements into a form that you call your own.

"You are intuitively aware that you form your image, and that you are independent of it. You do not realize

that you create your larger environment and the physical world as you know it by propelling your thoughts and emotions into matter – a breakthrough into three-dimensional life."[40]

26. A few health-related quotes from Abraham

"There is not a source of not Well-being. There is not a source of sickness. There is just the disallowance of wellness. In every particle of the Universe there is that which is wanted and lack of it."[41]

~

"Anything you see anyone experiencing, that is a diminishment of wellbeing, always at the root of it is resistance – there's no question about it."[42]

~

"Someone needs to be healed – states are just a snapshot of how other people have handled energy. It doesn't matter what a situation is, it can be aligned."[43]

~

"The situation isn't the reason I feel this way; my focus is the way I feel this way."[44]

~

"Any malady in your physical body was a lot longer in coming than it takes to release it."[45]

~

"Someone asked us [recently], 'Is there any limitation to the body's ability to heal?' And we said, 'None, other than the belief that you hold.' And he said, 'Then why aren't people growing new limbs?' And we said, 'Because no one believes that they can.'"[46]

27. Serving others at our own expense

We are often given the view that helping and being of service to others is of prime importance – regardless of our own needs. Abraham says that the universe is organised around 'alignment' and whilst it is sometimes a pleasure, or easy to assist someone, whilst still being in alignment with our true self, it should never be a case of 'should' or 'must'. Sometimes people become trapped in their feeling (or belief) that they always have to be available to others' needs, no matter what. This can cause such an inner conflict that the path of least resistance is to become ill, rather than to overtly withdraw your help. As Abraham says, it ends up where...

"You have to make yourself sick enough that that's the path of least resistance! Because service to others stands as paramount to all things."

Similarly, there are many instances where the perceived pain of changing a situation or behaviour feels worse than actually enduring an upset, or pain, that currently exists in your physical experience. A bit like saying you would rather walk in the rain than ask someone for the bus fare.

28. Reboot your health

Some years ago, I had a computer 'Netbook' – a small version of a 'laptop' – that could be easily transported around. However, it gradually seemed to slow down until, one day, it became virtually unusable. A search on the Internet reminded me that it contained its original program within a piece of memory that could not be erased, changed, or damaged. All I had to do was overwrite my existing situation by reloading its 'operating system' from this original program.

What if you could do the same with your health? What if, somewhere, there is a personal program connected to your physical expression? And what if you could reset even just some of your functionality, without erasing the bits you wish to keep?

Putting to one side conventional knowledge on such matters, let's be as children and pretend that anything is possible. Let's pretend that we are going to 'tune in to' our original health program; the bit that is labelled 'natural healthy state of being'. Now imagine that this is sending data to your DNA and genes – with instructions to repair any areas that have changed their nature from their original optimal performance. See if you can make up an imaginative image of this in your thoughts. What might it look like? How would it feel as you started to regenerate?

Let me remind you of the last two paragraphs of Seth quotes in section 25:

"Quite literally, the 'inner self' forms the body by magically transforming thoughts and emotions into physical counterparts. You grow the body. Its condition perfectly mirrors your subjective state at any given time. Using atoms and molecules, you build your body, forming basic elements into a form that you call your own.

"You are intuitively aware that you form your image, and that you are independent of it. You do not realize that you create your larger environment and the physical world as you know it by propelling your thoughts and emotions into matter – a breakthrough into three-dimensional life."

In other statements,[47] Seth informs us that our physical bodies are quite literally destroyed and rebuilt millions of times a second – that we do not preserve physical continuity from one moment to the next. If this is an inescapable universal truth of creative consciousness forming physical matter, mental transformations of energy by an entity into physical reality (or 'idea construction'[48], as Seth sometimes calls it) then the physical projection of our self must be both independent of, but also connected to, its projector. All personal experiences and memories must have some sort of two-way interaction between our inviolate source and our reconstructed physicality – giving the illusion of remembered and experienced linear continuity.

29. Thoughts can cause molecular changes to your Genes

A study undertaken by researchers in Wisconsin, Spain, and France, reported[49] the first evidence of specific molecular changes in the body following a period of intensive mindfulness practice.

"To the best of our knowledge, this is the first paper that shows rapid alterations in gene expression within subjects associated with mindfulness meditation practice.[50]

"Most interestingly, the changes were observed in genes that are the current targets of anti-inflammatory and analgesic drugs."[51]

Gene activity can change according to perception

According to Dr Bruce Lipton[52], gene activity can change on a daily basis. If the perception in your mind is reflected in the chemistry of your body, and if your nervous system reads and interprets the environment and then controls the blood's chemistry, then you can literally change the fate of your cells by altering your thoughts.

Dr Lipton's research demonstrates that by changing your perception, your mind can alter the activity of your genes and create over thirty thousand variations of products from each gene. He gives more detail by saying that the gene programs are contained within the nucleus of the cell, and you can rewrite those genetic programs through changing your blood chemistry.

Put simply, this means that we need to change the way we think if we are to heal conditions such as cancer.

"The function of the mind is to create coherence between our beliefs and the reality we experience," Dr Lipton said. *"What that means is that your mind will adjust the body's biology and behaviour to fit with your beliefs. If you've been told you'll die in six months and your mind believes it, you most likely will die in six months. That's called the nocebo effect, the result of a negative thought, which is the opposite of the placebo effect, where healing is mediated by a positive thought."*

That dynamic points to a three-party system: there's the part of you that swears it doesn't want to die (the conscious mind); trumped by the part that believes you will (the doctor's prognosis mediated by the subconscious mind); which then throws into gear the chemical reaction (mediated by the brain's chemistry) to make sure the body conforms to the dominant belief. (Neuroscience suggests that the subconscious controls 95 percent of our lives.)[53]

With a similar explanation to my 'reinstalling the computer program', and Seth's comment that, *the 'inner self' forms the body by magically transforming thoughts and emotions into physical counterparts'*, Dr Lipton asks rhetorically:

"Did I distort the original broadcast pattern? Absolutely not. The original pattern is there, but via the dials of adjustment, I can change the appearance of that pattern without changing the original broadcast."

30. Curing cancer

In addition to the aforementioned information, I would now like to mention three physical things that some believe can clear many disorders, including some cancers:

- Honey and cider vinegar[54]
- Cannabis or marijuana[55]
- Resonant frequencies[56]

Although I am not advocating any proof for the above, some of the information available on the Internet is certainly interesting and worth further exploration – particularly the use of sound. It may also be of interest to those of you whose current beliefs prefer to work within the realms of physical reality. It can also help some people to believe in the possibility of something and at the same time emphasise such a belief with a physical action to reinforce a mental expectation. You will in fact discover many 'cures for cancer' via the Internet and beyond. I'd suggest a large percentage of them are most unlikely, but having said this, if you find one that improves your condition, and you truly believe in it, then by all means use it. Do not however, expect it to be a cure-all for other people. Suggest it if you want to, but never advertise it as 'an amazing wonder cure', or pressure anyone into accepting your beliefs about reality as truths or facts.

I might suggest here, that if you are diagnosed with something, have a go at self-healing before deciding on only conventional medical remedies or surgery. That does not mean, that you might then move towards a more conventional approach and, in a way, you could say that as you are a 'spiritual being' in a physical reality, you have created in your reality, the physical help you require, at a physical level. There is nothing wrong in having a helping hand through what seems to be conventional means.

Alternative healing can work well, but many leave it as a last resort when medical interventions fail to work and by now, have caused additional imbalances that divert the body's resources and possibly, through those stresses, leave little apparent time for recovery.

31. Resistance stops receipt

Imagine a tug-of-war, where two opposing teams of equally matched individuals attempt to pull a rope marker across a line. This is how most people are with their visualisations. You want something... but then immediately start thinking of why you can't have it.

As well as the effect this can have on your ability with the Law of Attraction, it can also affect your potential to improve your health. The message we often send out in our vibration is: I want it, but I don't. I'd like it, but I can't have it because...

You might say you do not do that, but you still don't get the outcomes you desire. One reason for this is 'root assumptions'[57] or 'root beliefs'. Regardless of what you think about in this moment of 'now', you might have spent quite a while in your life believing that some things cannot happen, either because you have been told they cannot happen factually or scientifically, or because at some time or other, you have convinced yourself of their unlikeliness or impossibility – in your experience. So although you desire a change in your life, and are not consciously reflecting on the likely plausibility, something resides within your being that has a stronger, opposing belief than the one you are now focusing on. Therefore, your general vibration and frequency of output is of a fairly consistent nature, regardless of your inspired highs or desperate lows. What you are aiming for is a new consistency. You could call it your modus operandi or your normal knee-jerk reaction to events.

For example, your first reaction to any upsetting situation might be, 'it's a disaster!' With a more mindful awareness you may gradually change this and when you notice that your first reaction is closer to, 'that's okay – no need to give energy to this.' then you know you have changed.

There are a few things you can try out to develop this:

1. Write down the health you desire
2. Write down the reasons you want this
3. Write down the reasons you believe you will have this
4. Write down anything that might make this difficult
5. Write down any belief you have about any aspect of your desire and whether this belief

holds any truth. Seek the origin of the belief. Form a new, more helpful, belief to put in its place and then actively look for evidence of your new belief — as you have always done with your old one

6. Repeat the first 3 again

32. Request assistance

Sometimes it is difficult to know what to do; how to change something that you have experienced and believed in for a long time; or even know what to ask. Because it's not always easy to focus attention in the waking state, before you go to bed to sleep, send out the thought: I would like to gain clarity about... [*add here the thing you want clarity about*]. Try to keep your request simple.

Here are a few examples:

- I want clarity about my health
- I want help with my ability to focus my thoughts in more positive ways
- I wish to attract improvement in my health
- I want help and guidance to feel better

The request can be about anything, but keep it as clear as you can. You can repeat the same request as often as you like. You do not have to look for the answer. You will probably find that some new clarity just comes to you and it could be via any number of ways.

One thing I have noticed is that the universe will often deliver answers in ways that seem quite ordinary. A friend may send you a link to a website, or pass on a book to you containing the very information you have been asking about. You might overhear a conversation or see something written on a sign. You might be walking and suddenly a dog barks which triggers an idea in your mind. All these things seem quite ordinary and quite removed from the guru you were possibly expecting to see materialize in front of you. Many signs are symbolic rather than literal. Learn to be aware of symbolism and become open to its interpretation through your intuition. Practice noticing your regular thoughts around your health. Are they helpful or limiting? Can you counteract your response with a better feeling one? Try saying: 'I decide to be well from now on.'

I remember when I first noticed this ordinary feedback. I had reached a point where I felt I had all the information I now needed to progress my spiritual evolution. I wasn't particularly interested in other people recommending books and videos on subjects I already knew enough about, or that might detract from the focus I wanted to maintain. Sometimes I felt my ego prodding me with its annoyance. But gradually, it dawned on me that by accepting some of these recommendations, I was allowing the universe to give me a bit more information that I had been thinking about – something to build on my clarity.

Sometimes, you are the channel for someone else's clarity. The universe will use whatever means it has at its disposal – and usually takes the quickest and easiest route. (See next section).

33. Focusing attention

Abraham[58] encourages us to train ourselves to focus in a way that stimulates more positive feedback:

"We would demonstrate to everyone that we are cheerful, that we are optimistic, that we are happy, that we are looking for the best-feeling thought that we can find — and that we've practiced it so much that we often find it. And then, as people say to you, in accusing tones, 'Oh, you are a Pollyanna,' announce to them, 'Pollyanna lived a very happy life."[59]

Seth reminds us more bluntly that:

"You will react, [therefore,] to all the information that you receive according to your conscious beliefs concerning the nature of reality."[60]

He also talks about a time before our physical birth:

"Within the basic framework of the body chosen before physical birth, the individual has full freedom to create a perfectly healthy functioning form. The form is, however, a mirror of beliefs, and will accurately materialise in flesh those ideas held by the conscious mind.[61]

"That is one of the body's primary functions. A sick body is performing that function then, in its way, as well as a healthy one. It is your most intimate feedback system, changing with your thought and experience, giving you in flesh the physical counterpart of your thought. So it is futile to become angry at a symptom, or to deride the body for its condition when it is presenting you with the corporeal replica of your own thought, as it was meant to do."[62]

Seth offers us many pearls of wisdom and a depth of understanding that far surpasses most other knowledge available in our physical domain. Here is another quote taken from the same source:

"A man believing he has heart trouble will finally, through his own anxiety, affect the functioning of his 'involuntary' system until his heart is definitely harmed if the belief goes unchecked. The conscious mind directs the so-called involuntary systems of the body, and not the other way around... Once more, you will not be sick if you think you are well – but

there may be other ideas that make you believe in the necessity of poor health."[63]

So you can appreciate by now, the importance of recognising what you are placing your daily attention on. The first change towards renewing your health is to recognise the thoughts and feelings you have about your health and then to question their validity in the light of your new understanding.

I would add here, in the context of the above information, we must make more conscious decisions about the information we receive through social media, in fact, the media and news in general, and advertising (as mentioned above in section 8). Suggestions that worry us about our health and scaremongering such as, 'x number of people will get [enter here any health calamity of your choice]', is not helpful to either individual or collective well-being – regardless of any well-meaning intention.

34. Ho'oponopono

Ho'oponopono (*ho-o-pono-pono*) is an ancient Hawaiian practice of reconciliation and forgiveness which literally means, to 'make right'. It is also referred to as 'SITH' (Self Identity Through Ho'oponopono) by its originator in this form, Morrnah N Simeona and subsequently taught by former clinical psychologist, Dr Ihaleakala Hew Len (who had successfully used the 'cleaning' techniques in a Hawaiian State Hospital for mentally ill criminals).

I first came across Ho'oponopono via a friend. As it wasn't something that immediately grabbed my interest at the time, I passed the information on to another friend who I thought might be interested. She in turn decided to travel to Hawaii to discover more, and attended a course led by Dr Hew Len. After seeing how using Ho'oponopono rapidly changed some difficult circumstances in my friend's life, I decided to take another look at it myself. To my surprise, it seemed to improve any situation I directed my attention towards, whilst reciting an associated mantra (see below).

The basic premise of Ho'oponopono is linked to this question that Dr Hew Len says we must ask ourselves when faced with any situation or circumstance that we would rather change:

**What is it within me
that is attracting this situation?**

The power of this question resides in each individual accepting full responsibility for everything that comes into his, her, their, personal life awareness. Dr Hew Len realised that for mentally ill criminals to show up in his life, he had to be, at some level, creating them. By 'cleaning' on and healing his own thoughts and feelings, he gradually saw those same people leaving his experience – very often by recovering, or sometimes being transferred to other accommodation, until eventually, his Hospital Ward was closed. (This example also relates to what I mentioned earlier about many things in our world being opposite to what we think they are. Often in our physical experience, it is the [feedback] symptom we see and react to – not the cause).

Bear in mind that Seth and Abraham (previously mentioned) inform us that every individual creates their own reality. Once you accept this, the Hew Len question makes complete sense. It links directly to the law of attraction, personal beliefs, and expectations. The basic mantra is:

I'm sorry
Please forgive me
I love you
Thank you

Simply recite the mantra inside your head. The order of the first three isn't important and personally, I have found this works well...

I love you
I'm sorry
Please forgive me
Thank you

(My suggestion is that if you find it hard to begin with 'I love you' it's possibly easier to start with 'I'm sorry').

There is much more to Ho'oponopono than I have picked out for attention, for those who wish to explore it more fully, but for my purposes and understanding, what has been provided here is all that you need to get started. No explanation of why this is so effective is necessary to understand for it to work, but if you want to know more, just look it up online. All you have to do is keep repeating the mantra over and over, whilst holding any thought, or emotion, in your mind that you wish to clean. Once you start, you will probably find that more thoughts and their associated feelings surface for cleaning. Just keep going until it feels comfortable to stop. Use the mantra as often as you like. One thing you will notice is that the strength of your upset or negativity will subside after using the mantra a few times. The main thing is to remember to use it. Don't treat it like a sandwich toaster – using it every day for a week, putting it away in the cupboard and suddenly rediscovering it a year later.

35. Understanding deliberate creation

Every time you have a thought about something, there is a 'probable outcome' associated with that action. Depending on your focus, some probabilities become more likely to manifest than others – but all exist together. Remember the well-known saying: 'Where attention goes, energy flows.'[64]

Although I wrote a booklet called 'Deliberate Creation – a pocket guide to successful manifesting', the principles of this can equally be applied to good health and being well. You have to know that you have a choice, no matter how things may appear to you in your immediate experience. Remember that what you perceive as the present is actually the feedback of your last action – not your current one.

36. Exercises

Over the next couple of pages are a few exercises and mental processes that you can practice to improve or maintain your good health. Feel free to pick and choose – you do not have to do all of them at once. At first, some of these will demand something of a leap of faith and a level of trust that may seem contrary to how you feel. But keep going. Much of our behaviour is habitual and within the boundaries of our comfort levels – and what we have previously decided is true in our experience.

1. Acknowledge your responsibility for your own wellbeing. Accept that you alone are responsible for your life and circumstances and because of this, you have the power

within you to change any aspect of your life –
if you so choose

2. Every day, decide that your body is always
   acting on your behalf to restore healthy
   balance

3. Every night before sleeping, ask the cells of
   your body to restore your health in specific
   areas

4. Know that you can be well or know that your
   health can improve and is improving

5. Remember that what you witness in your
   health today is what you created previously.
   Because you created your condition, you can
   change it

6. Breathe in slowly through the nose. As you
   breathe out slowly through the mouth, send
   all of your healing thoughts to an area that
   you wish to receive healing energy

7. Imagine bright, morning sunlight shining on
   your head – or better still, stand outside in
   sunlight – and imagine sending that light to
   any area where you wish for healing to occur

8. Ask out loud: 'How can my health get any
   better than this?'

9. Create a daily practice for at least a full
   month. Leave yourself a reminder note where
   you will see it every day. Or if you have a
   mobile, work with a friend so that one of you
   always remembers to text the other a
   reminder word such as, 'focus'.

37. Summary and final thoughts

Let's overview some of the things contained in this book and mix in a few other thoughts:

- Your natural state is one of good health, until something within you causes a resistance
- What you focus your attention on becomes stronger and may eventually gain form in your physical experience
- Watching or listening to other people's opinions about health – particularly through advertising, is not helpful if it causes you to feel fearful
- Emotions are a powerful motivator and can affect your body chemistry in positive or negative ways
- Beliefs about our lives are not facts that cannot be changed or modified
- Time is not what it seems. You do not have to wait to feel better
- Ask yourself: 'Why am I unwell?' Quickly, what answer comes to you first?
- Decide to change your own beliefs about health from negative to positive. Reboot your wellbeing
- You can decide to feel better about any situation you experience. This will take practice and often [to begin with] go against rational thought or physical feedback

- To make a change in a habit, or to form a new habit, you probably need to practice every day for up to a month. If you miss a day – start again.
- Consciously feel good about as many things as you can on a daily basis to get into the practice of expecting better outcomes
- Ask aloud: 'How can my life get any better than this? What else is possible for my good health [or recovery]?'
- Get into a habit of thinking about best-case scenarios
- Think about solutions rather than problems
- Try to mentally relax more. Spend less time focusing on health worries and stop getting cross with yourself for not being able to get better. Acknowledge if you have to, that you do not know how to get better, but that your body will instinctively know what to do if you get out of the way.
- Do not decide that there are only certain ways for things to happen. Always leave room for something unexpected that may never have occurred to you
- Avoid watching negative current affairs, news, soaps, and negatively biased TV reality shows, etc. – you want to feel better, not worse.
- Avoid negative posts on social media, and avoid adding to conflict or getting into arguments

- Be mindful of your self-talk when alone and the things you say in conversation with others
- If you hear yourself saying, or agreeing with, something out of habit, ask yourself if it is really true for you – perhaps you want to change that old belief
- Be mindful of the judgements you make in relation to others – you're only judging yourself. Their actions in your experience are only feedback to your inner output
- Other people's [sometimes challenging] reactions to you are your personal feedback – not a personal attack
- Emotional feelings that you have are your inner guidance system – act on them
- Keep a little notebook and write down any inspired thoughts you have but may not wish to act on immediately – and periodically look through it
- Again, realise that all physical reality is only personal feedback for you – if you want to know what your vibrational output is like, simply observe what is around you in your daily experience
- Offer gratitude as often as you can and thank whatever feedback comes your way
- Try out Ho'oponopono to see if you can change a situation for the better

- Desire with emotion and positive expectation, but with no attachment to outcome. Dream more – day as well as night
- Develop the feeling of *knowing* that everything will turn out for the best and highest good of everyone – including you
- Accept that everyone is doing their best with whatever they have access to
- Nothing is so important that you need to be anxious about it – imagine looking at the Earth from space, before zooming back in on the little bit of physical stuff that is your world
- Buy yourself an 'Easy button' – press it every time something positive happens with little effort on your part and listen to it say, 'That was easy!'
- If the only time you can make a difference is in every moment of 'now', actively decide on as many desirable things as possible
- Start writing down positive things in your new life of being well, as if they exist now. It's a great way to focus your attention long enough to let Law of Attraction kick in – which according to Abraham starts at only 17 seconds, but is equivalent to 2000 hours of physical action. And once you reach 68 seconds, Abraham says that this is equivalent to about 2 million action hours
- The universe is a safe place if you allow it to be. Experiment with trusting the universe

- Always intend to do what you enjoy most
- Watch a film, or listen to some audio, that causes you to laugh out loud and feel good
- Pay attention to how you feel – not just in the moment, but over a period of time
- Make a little chart with lines of scales for each day of a month, from 0 to 10 and each day put a circle around a number, where 0 is lower energy or negative feeling and 10 is higher energy and feeling great! See if you notice an overall improvement as you go on

A last word from Seth:

"You must realize that you do create your own reality because of your beliefs about it. Therefore, try to understand that the particular dilemma or illness is not an event forced upon you by some other agency.

"Realize that to some extent or another your dilemma or your illness has been chosen by you and that this choosing has been done in bits and pieces of small, seemingly inconsequential choices.

"Each choice, however, has led up to your current predicament, whatever its nature."[65]

A last word from Abraham:

"Resistance is about believing that you are vulnerable or susceptible to something not wanted and holding

a stance of protection – which only holds you in a place of not letting in the Well-being that would be there otherwise. There is nothing big enough to protect you from unwanted things, and there are no unwanted things big enough to get into your experience."[66]

A last word from Richard:

"Know that anything is possible! If you can imagine it – you can manifest it."

Appendix

[1] www.masaru-emoto.net/english/water-crystal.html

[2] Self-talk is the act or practice of talking to oneself, either aloud or silently and mentally.

[3] Max Gerson (1881-1959) was a German-born American physician who developed the Gerson Therapy - a plant-based and entirely organic, dietary-based alternative cancer treatment that he claimed could cure cancer and most chronic, degenerative diseases. It is essentially based around the daily juicing of about 15-20 pounds of organically-grown fruits and vegetables. In fact, the Gerson Institute's recommended intake is up to one glass every hour, up to 13 times per day. See: http://gerson.org and http://gerson.org/gerpress/the-gerson-therapy Dr Max Gerson's daughter, Charlotte Gerson, founded the current Gerson Institute in 1977, to spread awareness of the Gerson Therapy.

[4] GP (General Practitioner – a UK term for a physician who is not a specialist but treats all illnesses)

[5] Research: Men's Health Forum (MHF) has found that men in Britain go to the doctors 20% less than women.

[6] Seth is a non-physical energy personality – channelled by Jane Roberts between the 1960s and 1980s whose vast commentary, teachings, and insights on the nature of personal reality were noted down by Jane's partner, Rob Butts and published in several books (still available).

[7] Op. cit. Law of Attraction

[8] You may have to search for material in support of this claim, but one place I discovered is www.radicalremission.com

[9] 'Snake oil' originally referred to fraudulent health products or unproven medicine but has come to refer to

any product with questionable or unverifiable quality or benefit.

[10] Whilst I may talk in terms of a personal vibrational frequency, I believe that Seth (see previous) refers to the same as 'feeling-tones'. Our vibrational frequency is transmitted all around us – first as consciousness units (CUs) and then as electromagnetic energy (EE) units and these interface with the 'All That Is' consciousness (which is the creator of our universe and the physical framework we experience on Earth).

[11] Op. cit. Seth

[12] Samuel Langhorne Clemens (1835-1910), better known by his pen name Mark Twain, was an American author and humourist.

[13] (Physiology) relating to, or controlled by, the autonomic nervous system – 'autonomic reflexes'

[14] Dr Hasmukh Joshi, vice-chair of the Royal College of GPs.

[15] The notion of 'virus' used here is because it is a quote – not necessarily a truth in every reality.

[16] RG author comment

[17] The National Pure Water association

[18] In areas of the world where fluoride is added to drinking water it is hydrofluoric acid which is a compound of fluorine that is a chemical by-product of aluminium, steel, cement, phosphate, and nuclear weapons manufacturing. Hydrofluoric acid is used to refine high octane gasoline, to make fluorocarbons and chlorofluorocarbons for freezers and air conditioners, and to manufacture computer screens, fluorescent light bulbs, semiconductors, plastics, herbicides, and toothpaste. Fluorosilicic acid is a waste product of the phosphate fertilizer industry and is heavily contaminated with toxins

and heavy metals (including the cancerous arsenic, lead and cadmium) and radioactive materials. This substance is the waste residue from the superphosphate fertilizer industry.

[19] RMS Titanic was a British passenger liner that sank in the North Atlantic Ocean in April, 1912 after colliding with an iceberg during her maiden voyage from Southampton, UK, to New York City, US.

[20] Op. cit. Seth

[21] Seth: The Nature of Personal Reality, Session 609 – The Manufacture of Personal Reality.

[22] Vibrational resonance in this context could be described as the matching of something given off by one thing being sympathetically received by another of a similar disposition.

[23] Abraham is a collective of teachers channelled by Esther Hicks. See www.abraham-hicks.com

[24] Op. cit. Abraham

[25] A tuning fork is an acoustic resonator in the form of a two-pronged fork with the prongs (tines) formed from a U-shaped bar of elastic metal (usually steel). It resonates at a specific constant pitch when set vibrating by striking it against a surface or with an object, and emits a pure musical tone after waiting a moment to allow some high overtones to die out. The pitch that a particular tuning fork generates depends on the length and mass of the two prongs. It is frequently used as a standard of pitch to tune musical instruments.

[26] Op. cit. Seth

[27] The spacious present is the truth of our situation – where there is no real past or future and no real distance to travel. For fuller explanations from Seth, go to www.sethnet.org where my friend, Lynda Madden Dahl,

carefully curates all of the Seth material, or www.nirvikalpa.com where you can search Seth quotes.

[28] Seth refers to the multidimensional nature of personalities throughout his works but broadly talks of: '...the soul or overall individual identity, the true multidimensional self.' – Seth Speaks Session 538

[29] Seth says that '...Within the moment point, the smallest thought is brought to fruition, the slightest possibility explored, the probabilities thoroughly examined, the least or most forceful feeling entertained. It is difficult to explain this clearly, and yet the moment point is the framework within which we have our psychological experience.' – Seth Speaks, Session 514

[30] Behaviour covers both physical and emotional action.

[31] Emotional origins can sometimes be multi-layered.

[32] Newtonian refers to the work of Isaac Newton

[33] Newton's third law is: For every action, there is an equal and opposite reaction.

[34] Reincarnation is the belief that after death, we can be reborn into a new physical body and have a new life.

[35] The Quantum Universe simply put: Everything that can happen does happen.

[36] Lynda Madden Dahl is an author of several books including, 'Living a Safe Universe', based on Seth's teachings.

[37] The Three Creative Dilemmas are beyond the scope of this booklet, but Seth says: 'These dilemmas represent three areas within which inner reality, or inner vitality, can experience itself.' And he adds the creative dilemmas are the basis for all realities, and the heart of all meaning.

[38] Immersive gaming: A perception of being physically present in a non-physical world

[39] Remember what I said about soul-searching in section 22.

[40] Seth Speaks, Session 520

[41] Excerpted from the workshop: Syracuse, NY on October 17, 1996

[42] Jerry Hicks asks Abraham a question about Esther's health (Circa 2007)

[43] Originally from a YouTube clip 'What needs healing most in the human species?'

[44] Op.cit. YouTube clip

[45] Abraham – Napa, CA, February 27, 1997

[46] Abraham – San Rafael, CA on February 27, 1999

[47] Information in other Seth books

[48] First written down by Jane Roberts and forerunner to the Seth Material (Circa 1963)

[49] First reported publicly around 2013-14 and the study published in the Journal, Psychoneuroendocrinology.

[50] Richard J Davidson, founder of the Centre for Investigating Healthy Minds and the William James and Vilas Professor of Psychology and Psychiatry at the University of Wisconsin-Madison.

[51] Perla Kaliman, first author of the article and a researcher at the Institute of Biomedical Research of Barcelona, Spain (IIBB-CSIC-IDIBAPS).

[52] Dr Bruce H Lipton, PhD is an internationally recognized leader in bridging science and spirit. He also uses the term: EpiGenetics. www.brucelipton.com

[53] Original source articles from news.wisc.edu/22370 and brucelipton.com

[54] Honey has many historically mentioned curative properties and the use of vinegar (acetate) of any kind has proven to be beneficial for several health-related

improvements, including the alleviation of Gout. See: www.handoflight.org/gout (article by George Glasser)

[55] The use of certain plant drugs to improve difficult health conditions is gradually becoming increasingly well-documented and more publically accepted as having validity in helping a range of illnesses including Alzheimer's.

[56] Anthony Holland, a composer and electronic musician at Skidmore College in Saratoga Springs, NY, has developed an idea of bombarding cancer cells with electromagnetic waves to remove them. You can see his TEDx lecture here: www.handoflight.org/cancer

[57] Root assumptions represent the basic premises upon which a given existence-system is formed.
Seth - The Early Sessions

[58] Op. cit. Abraham

[59] Excerpted from: Atlanta, GA on April 28, 2005

[60] The Nature of Personal Reality, Session 617 (1972)

[61] Seth has also mentioned in other books, that we hold our beliefs through physical transition and this doubtless works in both directions of the birth and death cycle.

[62] The Nature of Personal Reality, Session 626 (1972)

[63] Ibid.

[64] Attributed to James Redfield, author of The Celestine Prophecy.

[65] The Way Toward Health, Chapter 8

[66] Excerpted from the workshop: Atlanta, GA, 4 November, 2000

www.ingramcontent.com/pod-product-compliance
Lightning Source LLC
Chambersburg PA
CBHW022128280326
41933CB00007B/588